Ülvan Özad

Intervertebral Disc: Anatomy, Materials and Design

Ülvan Özad

Intervertebral Disc: Anatomy, Materials and Design

LAP LAMBERT Academic Publishing

Impressum / Imprint

Bibliografische Information der Deutschen Nationalbibliothek: Die Deutsche Nationalbibliothek verzeichnet diese Publikation in der Deutschen Nationalbibliografie; detaillierte bibliografische Daten sind im Internet über http://dnb.d-nb.de abrufbar.

Alle in diesem Buch genannten Marken und Produktnamen unterliegen warenzeichen-, marken- oder patentrechtlichem Schutz bzw. sind Warenzeichen oder eingetragene Warenzeichen der jeweiligen Inhaber. Die Wiedergabe von Marken, Produktnamen, Gebrauchsnamen, Handelsnamen, Warenbezeichnungen u.s.w. in diesem Werk berechtigt auch ohne besondere Kennzeichnung nicht zu der Annahme, dass solche Namen im Sinne der Warenzeichen- und Markenschutzgesetzgebung als frei zu betrachten wären und daher von jedermann benutzt werden dürften.

Bibliographic information published by the Deutsche Nationalbibliothek: The Deutsche Nationalbibliothek lists this publication in the Deutsche Nationalbibliografie; detailed bibliographic data are available in the Internet at http://dnb.d-nb.de.

Any brand names and product names mentioned in this book are subject to trademark, brand or patent protection and are trademarks or registered trademarks of their respective holders. The use of brand names, product names, common names, trade names, product descriptions etc. even without a particular marking in this works is in no way to be construed to mean that such names may be regarded as unrestricted in respect of trademark and brand protection legislation and could thus be used by anyone.

Coverbild / Cover image: www.ingimage.com

Verlag / Publisher:
LAP LAMBERT Academic Publishing
ist ein Imprint der / is a trademark of
OmniScriptum GmbH & Co. KG
Heinrich-Böcking-Str. 6-8, 66121 Saarbrücken, Deutschland / Germany
Email: info@lap-publishing.com

Herstellung: siehe letzte Seite /
Printed at: see last page
ISBN: 978-3-659-53779-0

TABLE OF CONTENTS

I would like to dedicate this book to the greatest engineer I have ever known.

To My Father...

The Anatomy, Function and Diseases

Vertebral column is a vertical axis between the cranium and pelvis. There are 33 vertebral bones present in the spine. 24 vertebral bones are named as true vertebrae. These are able to perform movement and contain fibrocartillage in between. The most inferior 9 vertebral bones are the false vertebrae. Fusion between the bones leads to a fixed structure and prevents the movement except between sacrum and coccyx.[1] There are 5 parts: 7 cervical, 12 thoracic, 5 lumbar, 5 sacral (fused) and 4 coccygeal (fused) vertebrae in the direction of superior to inferior in vertebral column.[4]

In the cervical vertebrae, bilateral foramens are present for the passage of vertebral artery towards the brain. The most superior, first cervical vertebra is named as atlas and it possesses facets for articulating with the occipital condyle of the skull and the axis. Second cervical vertebra, axis, involves a projection named as the odontoid process (dens) and this articulates with atlas and facets. The fused sacral bones form sacrum which articulates with the most inferior lumbar vertebra superiorly, with pelvic bones laterally and the coccyx, which is formed by the coccygeal vertebra, inferiorly.[2]

Vertebral column is bent in certain directions to generate curvatures. The anteriorly convex curves resulting in bending forward are developed in foetal stages, from embryological outline, to take up less space in uterus, and these are named as the primary curvatures. Thoracic and sacral curvatures are primary curvatures. The secondary curvatures are anteriorly concave and they

3

develop throughout the growth of human beings in order to create a straight vertical axis for gravity and weight balance. The cervical curvature is created by holding the head up and the lumbar curvature is created by standing up.[3]

There are various typical characteristics present in all vertebrae. Anteriorly, the vertebral body which is the main weight bearing part of vertebra supporting the weight of more superior regions is present in various sizes and dimensions changing with the location, and getting gradually larger in inferior regions of the true vertebrae.[5,6]

Vertebral foramen is present in the vertebral arch for protecting the spinal cord and the blood supply. Transverse processes are raised from the merging points of pedicles and laminae and together with spinous processes, they act as sites for attachment of muscles and ligaments for assisting movement. Articular processes articulate between the adjacent vertebrae to prevent movement by zygapophyseal joints.[2,5] Anterior to the vertebral bodies, anterior longitudinal filament and in the vertebral canal, posterior longitudinal ligament lengthen through the whole vertebral column.

Vertebral column has numerous functions, mainly for providing protection and movement to the body. The most obvious function is the maintenance of the posture. It sustains the supporting of intrinsic and extrinsic back muscles where intrinsic muscles assist movement of individual vertebra and extrinsic muscles aid movement of the ribs and upper limbs.[3] Vertebral column protects the spinal cord which carries nerves between central nervous system and peripheral nervous system through passing the canal formed by foramina of vertebrae.

4

The pedicles lead to creation of intervertebral foramina which allows passage of spinal nerves, blood vessels and lymphatics. Presence of large number of vertebral bones articulating with each other offers movement to the vertebral column together with holding the skull and the intervertebral discs in between these bones provide shock-absorption for mainly protecting the central nervous system and brain. Thoracic vertebra is the axial skeleton present in the thorax, holding limbs and thoracic cage in place and it articulates with the ribs of thorax to provide movement in respiration. [2]

Individual vertebrae perform a limited movement in between them; however, the vertebral column as a whole can perform flexion, extension, lateral flexion and rotation movements. Cervical and the lumbar regions are the most flexible areas.[2] In the cervical region, atlas rotating around the dens projection of axis leads to rotation of the head.

The ranges of motion for cervical spine are 50° flexion, 45° lateral flexion, 80° rotation and 60° extension. In the lumbar region, due to the orientation of articular facets, rotatory movements are absent. The ranges of motion for lumbar vertebrae are 60° flexion, 25° lateral flexion and 25° extension.[29]

Spinal cord is a cylindrical bundle comprising of long nerves encircled by meninges and the cerebrospinal fluid, passing through the vertebral canal. It is part of the central nervous system, superiorly having medulla oblongata as continuation and inferiorly ending around the inferior border of most superior lumbar vertebra (L1). Below the spinal cord, there is cauda equina present up to the starting point of coccyx.

5

The height of spinal cord varies in correlation with the height of people, in a male with average height, it is 45cm.[2] 31 pairs of nerves passing from the spinal cord are present in five different areas of the vertebral column: 8 cervical, 12 thoracic, 5 lumbar, 5 sacral and 3 coccygeal (three segments merging into one nerve). When a lumbar puncture is applied, it is performed on below the level of second lumbar vertebra to prevent damaging the spinal cord.

The spinal cord is separated into two sections by anteriorly median fissure and posteriorly posterior median septum. There is grey matter in the centre which is surrounded by the white matter. Grey matter consists of sensory, connector and lower motor neurones. White matter has anterior, lateral and posterior columns, carrying sensory, connector and motor nerve fibres.[2]

Intervertebral discs unite the bodies of adjacent vertebrae and assist the formation of the gross vertebral column structure together with the ligaments except for coccyx and between the atlas and axis.[9] There are 24 intervertebral discs present.[16] They occupy approximately one fourth of the vertebral column length. In the evening, due to the weight applied on the intervertebral discs throughout the day, the height of people gets roughly two centimetres shorter compared to the morning. Since pedicles provide passage to the spinal nerves these are not joined by intervertebral discs.

There is no vascular blood supply to the discs and they obtain nutrients by diffusion from the hyaline cartilage end plates of adjacent vertebrae. The intervertebral disc cells are mainly anaerobic, producing lactic acid as a waste product.[16]

Histologically, intervertebral disc pads are formed by white fibrocartillage which is a tough and relatively inflexible structure containing white fibres and widely scattered cells embedded in a solid matrix with a gel-like core.[2] Fibrocartilage present in the intervertebral disc is one of the three types of cartilage: hyaline, elastic and fibrocartillage.

The specific cells making up cartilage, chondrocytes, also produce the matrix and fibres.[65] In body, fibrocartillage is seen in the areas of high stress, and has lower mechanical properties compared to hyaline. Collagen present provides the strength, elastic and shock-absorbing properties. The chondrocytes are originated from the mesenchymal stem cells.[64] The surrounding outer layer, annulus fibrosus is made from fibrocartillage in circular orientation of lamellae. It contains type 1 collagen.

Longitudinal ligament is anteriorly attached to the annulus fibrosus for supporting the structure and providing rigidity.[5] The core in the middle, nucleus pulposus is a fibrogelatinous, relatively softer semi-fluid structure, high in water content due to high proteoglycan (particularly aggrecan) amount present. Also, type 2 collagen and elastin are present in this part. Aggrecan and collagen are important in compression resistance.[66] Through ageing, the water content of nucleus pulposus decreases. There is no nociceptive innervation in the nucleus pulposus.[10]

The thickness of the intervertebral discs vary with the weight applied on the area they are present. They are thin in the superior regions and get increasingly thicker towards inferior regions, being thickest in the lumbar region except for the cervical region which also has thick intervertebral discs. Thick intervertebral presence provides more flexibility and ranges of movement to the cervical and lumbar regions.[6]

Size of a typical intervertebral disc in lumbar region has 45 millimetres anteroposterior width, 64 millimetres lateral width and 11 millimetres thickness.[16] Their shock-bearing characteristic and cartilaginous joint nature have an influence in increasing the flexibility and stability functions of the vertebral column.[5]

The load bearing function of spine and intervertebral discs are dependent on age, weight and physical activity of the people. The stress on the spine under normal pathological conditions could vary from 0.1 MPa (lying on prone position) to 2.3 MPa (carrying 20kg weight when spine is flexed back) and the normal standing upright position is approximately 0.5 MPa. [12,13,14,15] This stress is not equally distributed throughout the spine. Curvatures of the spine result in uneven distribution of stress in both vertical and horizontal axes.

Degeneration of vertebrae and intervertebral discs are therefore caused by the application of large, demanding repetitions of heavy weights on the areas receiving more stress.

Posterior annulus fibrosus is affected from this procedure to a large extent. This leads to load relocation from nucleus pulposus to posterior annulus fibrosus. The width of posterior annulus fibrosus increases by approximately 80%

together with decreasing height, leading to an increase in the stress experienced by 160%.[15]

There is nociceptive innervation in annulus fibrosus causing the feeling of pain. This procedure becomes worse by the increased age due to the decrease of bone density in vertebra and decreased water content in intervertebral disc by roughly 50%.[15] Vibrations and smoking are also harmful and can cause degenerative conditions.

Deformation of vertebrae and intervertebral discs could lead to nervous problems and back pain, affecting the lives of people to a very large extent. Back pain is one of the most prevalent conditions experienced by every four out of five people in their lifetimes.[17]

Exaggeration of the vertebral column curvatures could be caused by congenital, traumatic and environmental factors.[1] Kyphosis is exaggeration of the thoracic curve, causing a hunchback appearance. Scoliosis is anomalous lateral curvature of vertebral column. Lordosis is increased curvature in the lumbar region, also named as swayback.[18] These shape differences on posture cause changes to distribution of stress, resulting in deformation and pain.

There will be bone remodelling in the areas of high stress resulting in a higher bone density in the areas of high stress and brittle bones with lower bone density in the areas getting low stress. Deformation of intervertebral discs could also cause the patient to obtain a new posture in order to prevent pain in damaged areas, causing these exaggerated curves to form.

In the conditions deforming the intervertebral disc, due to restricted space in the vertebral canal and conditions limiting this space like vertebral dislocation or fraction, intervertebral disc prolapse and tumours, possibly either nerves are damaged of the or blood vessels are blocked resulting in painful and ischemic circumstances.[2] Damaged intervertebral discs cannot bear compressive stress efficiently . Compressive stress through the distance along diameter of young, middle age and degenerating intervertebral discs is different.

Projection of the nucleus pulposus, sometimes together with posterior longitudinal ligament, into the neural canal as herniation through the weak, damaged annulus fibrosus because of deformation or abnormal loading is called an intervertebral disc prolapse.[18] Herniated disc and slipped disc are other names used for describing the intervertebral disc prolapse. Bone and disc diseases or degeneration can cause gradual nucleus pulposus protrusion leading to a prolapsed disc.

The most common site for this condition is the lumbar vertebrae due to increased weight bearing needs of the lumbar site. Midline disc herniations compress spinal cord whereas the one sided herniations compress the nerve roots. The outcomes of this condition are variable from local pain to paralysis, depending on the size and presence duration of the protrusion.[2] This condition starts with disc degeneration and can end up with sequestration.

The treatment could be only conservational measures if there is no damage, medications such as painkillers and muscle relaxants, physiotherapy or exercise. If no improvement is seen after six weeks, a surgical operation is preferred for cutting out of the prolapsed part.[20] In severe conditions, intervertebral disc replacement is required.

As the gelatinous interior of the intervertebral disc protrudes, compression is applied on the nerve roots leading to various symptoms such a pain, sensory or motor loss, tingling or pins and needles. Nerve compression in lumbar region due to intervertebral disc herniation is very common and is called "sciatica".

Osteoarthritis of spine results from degeneration of bone and cartilage connecting facet joints in posterior location. Inflammation and gradual erosion of the facet joints result in increasing friction and pain together with decreased flexibility and range of movement.

In the progression of this condition, osteophytes (bone spurs growing due to increased remodelling of the bone in an attempt to repair the damage and for stabilizing the destabilized joint due to deformation) grow on the areas of deformation and the size of the bone increases. In this degenerative condition, in terms of bone cells, osteoblast activity increases in an attempt to repair the deformed area. Also, subchondral sclerosis takes place. This can lead to spinal stenosis causing irritation and compression of the nerves.

When spinal osteoarthritis takes place in the lumbar region and results in morning stiffness, painful lower back or sacroiliac joint, it is called lumbosacral arthritis. Osteoarthritis of spine in the cervical region causing pain and stiffness in neck is named as cervical spondylosis.[21] The outcomes of these conditions could be parasthesiae, severe pain and other sensory conditions due to nerve compression. [22]

The treatment of spinal osteoarthritis involves various steps such as: medications including NSAIDS and analgesics, exercise, loss of weight, physiotherapy, temperature or hydro- therapy, TENS, massage and surgical operation for bracing as the final choice.

The degenerative and non-reversible nature of this condition would eventually one in three patients to lumbar laminectomy, spinal fusion or dissectomy resulting in fixation by metal screws.[23]

In the case of metal screw use to combine the vertebrae, the metal will stay in the body and by causing a change in the distribution of weight and stress on vertebrae, unwanted bone remodelling will take place leading to higher bone density in the areas experiencing high stress and lower bone density in the areas experiencing low stress. Posture changes and due to limitation of vertebral motion range; hence movement ability of the patient decreases. The metal screws will also cause pain and discomfort. The risk of infection due to placement of such a large material into the body is present.

A solution is needed where intervertebral disc is changed to maintain the passage of the nerves open and to prevent nerve compression. Operation for changing an individual intervertebral disc is less invasive. However, the risks such as early wearing and displacement are still present and in such cases, early revision would be needed. This replacement technique is a relatively fresh idea in the business of medical engineering and various new ideas are still under research.

The two most popular designs which received FDA approval and widely used are Charite (for use in lumbar vertebral region) and ProDisc (for use in both cervical and lumbar vertebral regions).[26] The properties, anatomy and function of vertebral bone, intervertebral disc and fibrocartillage are crucial for design of an intervertebral disc replacement device. The designed device must have properties and functions as close to the real structure as possible, at least better than the functioning in the pathological condition causing deformation.

Critical Design Parameters

In defining the parameters for designing a medical device, structure of biomaterials, properties needed for the device and biomechanics of the body should be considered. The table below (Table 1) describes the critical design parameters.

Table 1: Design Parameters and Definitions

Design Parameters	Definition
Weight Bearing Properties and Strength	The implant must be strong enough to bear the weight of the upper body This could be around 2.4 times of the bodyweight.[30] This can be 170 kilograms in a lumbar spine replacement of an obese person and can have additional forces applied on it. This property must withstand for a long time since the implant stays in the body. The designed product must have a strength of at least 2.5 MPa which is the maximum stress applied on spine.[16]
Size	The size of implant is critical as if the implant is larger than vertebra, it will cause nerve compression and if it is

	smaller, it will cause instability in movements. The size of an intervertebral disc has 45 millimetres width, 64 millimetres length and 11 millimetres thickness. The thickness of the device designed will be larger, several centimetres since vertebral bone height will be reduced as well for attaching the device and removing the damaged bone. [16]
Movement Flexibility	Flexion, extension, lateral flexion and rotation movements should be allowed by the implant, helping the patient to sustain an active life by not limiting the activities performed. For cervical vertebra these values are: 50° flexion, 45° lateral flexion, 80° rotation and 60° extension. For lumbar vertebra these values are: 60° flexion, 25° lateral flexion and 25° extension.[29]
Compression Rigidity	The spine bears a compressive force varied by movements; the implant must be rigid and not break by a compressive force of at 2.4 times higher than body weight.[30]
Cost	The selling price of the product must be less than the NICE guideline limit £30,000, inclusive of production cost, hospital/surgery fee, profit and any additional costs.[28]

Insertibility	The implant must be insertable by the surgeon and should be minimally invasive for reducing the complications. The operation for insertion of the designed device should not be longer than the predicted operation time for vertebral fusion which is 4 hours (and unsuccessful operation rate is 5-25% for this duration) in terms of not increasing the risks and complications.[31]
Sterilization	The implant must be durable to high temperatures and chemicals such as Hydrogen Peroxide for disinfection and sterilization. The designed device should be durable for 170° dry heating for one hour duration or 132° for 15 minutes.[32]
Biocompatibility	Effects of Body on Implant - The implant should be durable to Chloride. Corrosion resistance and non-degradation properties are also required.

Effects of Implant on Body- The implant should be inert, non toxic and must not cause any local or systemic inflammation in the human body, provoking tissue damage. Minimal trauma to the surrounding tissue is targeted. |

Attachment	There are various ligaments, muscles, nerves and blood vessels around the vertebrae. The attachments of the implant must avoid damaging or irritating these structures. Screws placed must not loosen in flexion and lateral flexion movements. The recovery from a vertebral surgical operation could take up to one year.
Durability	The implant will stay in the body and is expected to assist patient for the rest of patient's life so it needs to be durable and non-degradable. The parameter for the designed product is survival at least for 15 years before failing and needing a revision surgery.
Ductility	The implant will be subject to repetitive forces due to movements such as walking, sitting down or running. The implant must not break upon these repetitive forces. A negative Poisson's ratio would prevent bulging and extending of the material on to spinal cord due to compressive forces acting on it.[33]
Practicality	The implant designed must be practical to use, i.e. it needs to be inserted in a short time (around 4 hours), in case of failure, access to the device and revision option must be available, it must be visible in medical diagnostic devices such as x-ray in order to follow up the success of

	the surgery, it should not take up a large space in the body, however fill the space of the removed intervertebral disc; and, must not affect the balance, metabolism and movements.

Ligaments, attachment areas of muscles, retroperitoneal organs, spinous processes and most importantly spinal column are the structures around intervertebral discs, preventing access in surgery. Posterolateral region is the easiest access area to the intervertebral discs since they are closer to skin in that anatomical area, and this access region is preferred by some surgeons because of reduced tissue damage and traumatised area.

Sympathetic trunk, lymphatic trunk, azygos and hemizygos veins, great vessels and nerves and spinal cord are present in posteriolateral region. This causes anterior access to be a more preferable region for surgery. An incision from the abdomen is followed by accessing the area by moving the organs to sides. This situation restricts the options for design such as inability to use large screws, prevention of sharp-edge use and minimum biological reactivity.

Removal of intervertebral disc followed by the placement and fixation of the device has restrictions due to limitations in extensibility of vertebral column (because of strong ligaments and muscles holding vertebrae together and possible nerve damage in case of a stretch). Several discs could be replaced as well as one disc in the same operation.[34]

Use of intervertebral disc replacement instead of vertebral fixation significantly reduces the area exposed in operation, hence the trauma, infections and healing duration. Intervertebral disc replacement is a relatively new technology so there is lack of patient follow-up for suggesting a gold standard of years for revision surgery. A review study performed by AA Patel et al. described the need to revision surgery being correlated with the surgical technique used.[27]

In terms of sterilizability, autoclave sterilizers, using the steam as the main source of sterilization; or, if sensitivity to heat is present, hydrogen peroxide, silver, bleach and chemical sterilizers could be used. Hydrogen peroxide would also be used during the operation before the placement of implant in the body. Radiation sterilization is also used, especially in pharmaceutical industry.[43,44]

Materials Analysis

Cobalt-chromium alloys, titanium and titanium alloys, stainless steels, polyethylene, polyurethane and ceramics are the common materials under consideration for intervertebral disc replacement products.[35] Rubber also could be a suitable material in intervertebral disc replacement product for nucleus pulposus. In choosing a material, biocompatibility and strength of the material are crucial for success of the surgical operation. Severe diseases lead to surgery for intervertebral disc. Beside intervertebral disc, bone would be affected and the attachment of the product to the vertebra would be fixed onto bone due to damage and resurfacing of cartilage.

Human bone has 130 MPa strength, 17 GPa Young's Modulus and 1.8 gcm^{-3} density.[36] The elastic modulus of nucleus pulposus is 5.7KPa and for annulus fibrosus, this value is 75.8-110.7KPa.[58] The materials selected will be used as replacements for these structures both in terms of properties and function; so, these properties are crucial in material selection.

There are four types of Cobalt-chromium alloys listed in ASTM as suitable for implants: CoCrMo (cast), CoCrWNi (wrought), CoNiCrMo (wrought) and CoNiCrMoWFe (wrought); however, two common types, CoCrMo and CoNiCrMo are mostly preferred. CoCrMo alloy is castable and beside dental uses, it is used for many artificial joint replacement products. CoNiCrMo is wroughtable by forging and is mostly used as the stem in the replacement products of weight-bearing joints. The molybdenum addition increases the strength of the material and chromium addition amplifies corrosion resistance properties.[36,53] The chromium content of CoCrMo is 27-30 % whereas CoNiCrMo has 19-21% chromium causing it to be less corrosion resistant; on the other hand, molybdenum content of CoNiCrMo is 5-7% whereas it is 9-10.5% in CoNiCrMo causing this one to be stronger. CoCrMo and CoNiCrMo has relatively same wear resistances, however CoNiCrMo has advantage in long lasting products because ultimate tensile strength and fatigue resistance making this product more suitable for long term uses; also, the frictional features of CoCrMo are deprived.[36,54] The table below (Table 2) demonstrates the mechanical properties of these two alloys.

Table 2: Mechanical Properties of Cobalt-Chromium Alloys [36,37,38]

Material	Tensile Strength (MPa)	Yield Strength (MPa)	Elongation (%)	Reduction of Area (%)	Young's Modulus (GPa)	Fatigue Strength (MPa)
CoCrMo (F75)	655	450	8	8	230	310
CoNiCrMo (F562)	793-1793	240-1585	8-50	35-65	230	--

Under normal conditions, cobalt is poisonous to bone cells, especially osteoblasts. When it is a chromium alloy, this situation is tolerated by cells and no impact is seen on these cells. CoCrMo is used in Triumph[39] intervertebral disc replacement devices and CoNiCrMo is not currently used in any intervertebral disc replacement products. ProDisc which is one of the main intervertebral disc replacement products used, also has CoCrMo end plates.[46]

CoNiCrMo is not corrosion resistant and biocompatible enough, so it is not appropriate. CoCrMo, as a strong, corrosion resistant, inert and biocompatible material with a high strength and young's modulus[51], is a suitable material for the plates of an intervertebral disc replacement product.

Four grades of Titanium and Ti6Al4V are differentiated by their impurity contents. Titanium alloys could be made stronger by thermomechanical processing. Vanadium is crucial for stabilization of the "body centered cubic structure" by decreasing the temperature for transformation.[36,54] The iron and oxygen content increases simultaneously with the grade but carbon content is nearly constant in all grades. The mechanical properties of Titanium and Ti6Al4V are provided in the table below (Table 3).

Table 3: Mechanical Properties of Titanium Alloys [36,40]

Material	Tensile Strength (MPa)	Yield Strength (MPa)	Elongation (%)	Young's Modulus (GPa)	Reduction of Area (%)
Grade 1	240	170	24	110	30
Grade 2	345	275	20	110	30
Grade 3	450	380	18	110	30
Grade 4	550	485	15	110	25
Ti6Al4V	860	795	10	110	25

Titanium gains resistance to oxidation by an oxide layer formation on surface. In cemented replacements, titanium particles will be inevitably released into the prostheses and in some occasions, accumulation of debris caused by wear could cause tissue response and form a cyst. [36] In spine surgeries, titanium is used in Coflex interspinous device[41] and Pliviopore vertebral implant. [42]

Lightweight, low density, flexible and debris-forming structures of titanium are desirable properties for an implant design. However, vertebrae withstand repetitive load application and the plates used in the intervertebral disc replacement device also need to be able to endure application of load.

Flexion of the plates due to application of load will lead to loosening of the device, instability in vertebrae or compression of spinal cord, pain, reduced function, possible tissue response due to irritation, and need to a revision surgery. Cyst formation could lead to tumours and serious health problems. A material with higher density and more rigid structure would be more appropriate for stability of vertebrae and continuation of activities in daily life.

In the material class of stainless steel, vanadium steel is not used in medical implants due to low corrosion resistance. Addition of molybdenum and decrease of carbon content lead to production of 316L stainless steel which could be used in implants. Table below (Table 4) demonstrates the material properties of stainless steel 316L. Corrosion could take place in stainless steel implants under oxygen-depleted situations. Therefore, it is only suitable for temporary use, or fixations such as screws and nails. Methods for surface modification are adopted to overcome this problem.[36,54]

Stainless steel, particularly for corrosive problems, is not also preferred for the plates of the intervertebral disc replacement, however it could be a particularly good material for design of temporary products like screws to fix or prevent compartment syndrome in the site of surgical operation.

Table 4: Mechanical Properties of Stainless Steel [36,45]

Material	Ultimate Tensile Strength (MPa)	Yield Strength (MPa)	Elongation (%)	Young's Modulus (GPa)	Rockwell Hardness
316L Stainless Steel	485-860	172-690	12-40	200	95 HRB

Metals are preferred as plates of the design because they have high Young's Moduli, increased strength is available through alloying and processing, ductility allows stress redistribution; hence, breaking and cracking becomes harder. Metal end plates will be attached to vertebral bones and they will be exposed to repetitive loading over a long time in the human body. To prevent failure, instability and loosening, these properties are important. As a result of the material properties described above, CoCrMo gives the impression of the most suitable material for the metal plate.

Polyethylene has five common types: high density polyethylene, ultra high molecular weight polyethylene, low density polyethylene, linear low density polyethylene and very low density polyethylene. As the density of the polyethylene decreases, the branching in structure increases. This leads to more flexible products to be produced by polymers possessing lower densities and stronger, more rigid products to be produced by polymers with higher densities. Polyethylene groups with lower densities are mainly used in industrial and consumable products whereas polyethylene with higher densities is preferred in medical implants due to being stronger and more durable.

Ultra high molecular weight polyethylene is a linear thermoplastic which is mainly used in the implants of load bearing joints; hence, it could be a suitable product for intervertebral disc replacement. The Young's modulus for ultra high molecular weight polyethylene is 0.8-1.6 GPa[67], density is 0.94 gcm^{-3} and the strength is 30MPa.[36]

An ultra high molecular weight intervertebral disc replacement product with cobalt-chromium alloy end plates is designed and produced by ProDisc. Polyethylene materials with lower densities are not used in this design because intervertebral discs and vertebral bones are load bearing structures and these materials are not strong, rigid or durable enough. Ultra high molecular weight polyethylene has lower young's modulus and strength values compared to vertebral bone. Due to this reason, a metal is preferred as the major weight bearing part and the ultra high molecular weight polyethylene is chosen as the moving middle part.

Polyurethane thermosetting materials are strong, oil and chemical resistant so these materials are used for coating purposes. [36]

Rubbers, either silicone, natural or synthetic, are used in implant fabrication. Natural rubber is also found in blood so it is compatible with human blood. Properties and characteristics are largely variable with production method. Silicone rubber, with dimethyl siloxane mer units, is a rubber used in medical products. These rubbers could mix with other polymers as well. Cross linking of low molecular weight polyethylenes produce a material like rubber.[36] Acroflex 100 is an FDA approved intervertebral disc replacement product using silicone elastomer as the core inner material and titanium endplates.

Elastomers are viscoelastic and they have lower young's moduli compared to other polymers; however, their yield strain is high. In loading, this material can stretch up to 700% (8 times) the original length it has, and return to its original state in removal of the loading.[49]

Ultra high molecular weight polyethylene could be a good substitute for annulus fibrosus in the intervertebral disc replacement product because of the strength, rigidity, frictionless self lubricated surface and durability of the material. Moreover inertness would eliminate the risks of inflammation and tissue response; and self-lubrication, biocompatibility, flexibility and low friction surface allows movement and acts as shock absorber.[54]

Ultra high molecular weight polyethylene can assist the need for load bearing properties of intervertebral disc. It bears the repetitive loading that will be applied and it will not bulge out to compress the nerves. Silicone elastomer, due to its viscoelastic properties, could be an alternative for nucleus pulposus. Also, placement of elastomer material in an intervertebral disc replacement product will help the distribution of weight in vertebra evenly, preventing bone remodelling due to excessive stress on one particular area and will increase the flexibility, allowing the patient to perform daily movements without restrictions.

Because of the low friction coefficient and high strength compared to other polymers, despite the low Young's modulus, ultra high molecular weight polyethylene can imitate annulus fibrosus and perform shock absorbing function of the intervertebral disc. Also, viscoelastic silicone elastomer could take the role of nucleus pulposus and contribute to shock bearing and balance maintenance roles. Addition of this extra material acts as a cushion and could be useful in preventing vibration on impact and protecting the patient, especially from cranial conditions that could be caused by transmission of vibration.

Nontoxic, bio-functionally durable, biocompatible, non-inflammatory, non-carcinogenic and non-allergic ceramics are named as bioceramics and used in medical implants.[36] Ceramics are not like polymers and metals in the way that ceramics do not experience plastic shearing due to the ionic bonding present in their structure.[50] This property results in almost no creep and non ductility.

Despite their strong structure, ceramics are brittle and they do not tolerate stress well. Silicates, oxides, hydrides, carbides, sulphides and many other compound additions are present in ceramics. The main disadvantage of ceramics group is the vulnerability to cracks due to not undergoing plastic deformation. Stress concentration in the crack will lead to weakening and easier breaking of the ceramic part.

Due to the latter, the tensile strength of ceramics is very low in comparison to compressive strength.[36] Ceramics are also corrosion resistant. Ceramics are used as cervical cages for optimum fusion. An example is Scient'x cervical cage. Ceramics could be used as bone grafts and when used in intervertebral disc replacement, but additional fixation would be needed.[56]

Due to the risk of cracking in repetitive load bearing situations, and need for fixation which creates the need for a more invasive operation with more inflammation and trauma risk, ceramics are not usually preferred in intervertebral disc replacement devices.

In this particular intervertebral disc design, ceramics are used as lateral coating of the metal plate core to promote bone growth, create a clear circumference around the vertebra and prevent compression of nerves by metal at movement, reduce the contact area of metal with living tissue, and provide additional attachment for preventing the loosening and failure of the device. By attaching ceramics to the circumference, direct load application on the ceramic part is prevented so the cracking and breaking risk of the ceramic component is significantly reduced.

Tantalum is a flexible, corrosion resistant and biocompatible metal that could be used as a porous inlay for enabling ingrowths of bone to constitute secondary stability.[53]

All of the materials described above are used in medical devices and manufacturing and processing of all materials are available in numerous

28

medical engineering companies. None of them requires an exceptionally specific device or skill for insertion, pre-operative procedure or fixation that a neurosurgery consultant cannot perform. The design that will be created would be insertible by the surgeon.

Ceramics and metals have better thermal and chemical stability compared to polymers; hence, they are easily sterilized by common sterilization techniques such as dry heat (160-190°C) and autoclave (steam sterilization).[57]

Rubber could be sterilized by dry heat. Polymer sterilization needs to be performed at lower temperatures, however due to presence of water vapour, steam sterilization (125-130°C and high pressure), radiation sterilization (manipulates structure to a brittle state) and high temperatures could not be used, so chemical agents like ethylene oxide or propylene oxide gases for a short duration (overnight) could be used instead.

Therefore, all materials that will be used in the experiment will be capable of undergoing a sterilization process that will significantly decrease infection and tissue response risk.

Design

The designed intervertebral disc replacement prosthesis involves superior and inferior parts. At each part, cobalt chromium alloy (CoCrMo) metal endplates are present. CoCrMo is chosen due to strength, corrosion resistance, wear resistance and biocompatibility. This CoCrMo metal core is surrounded by silicate ceramics which attach to CoCrMo plate with toothed junctions to enhance bone reformation and to create a bone- bone graft interphase for stimulation of bone grafts and additional strength to the prosthesis-bone attachment. After bone growth, this attachment will be strong and will prevent loosening of the material.

Ceramics part is not placed in a weight bearing place so there is no problem associated with its brittle nature. It surrounds the metal so it reduces the contact of metal with body, and diminishes the corrosion, inflammation and tissue response risks. The anteroposterior coronal section of the design is shown in the figure below (Figure 1). The attachment to bone is mainly performed by the triangular and the medial cross-shaped projections as demonstrated in the figure below by detailed and superoinferior transverse images (Figure 2).

The measurement values were designed according to the size of an intervertebral disc and vertebral bone. In the attachment of the device, the intervertebral disc and pathological cartilage will be removed, leaving resurfaced bone as attachment site.

Figure 1: Metal and Ceramic Plate

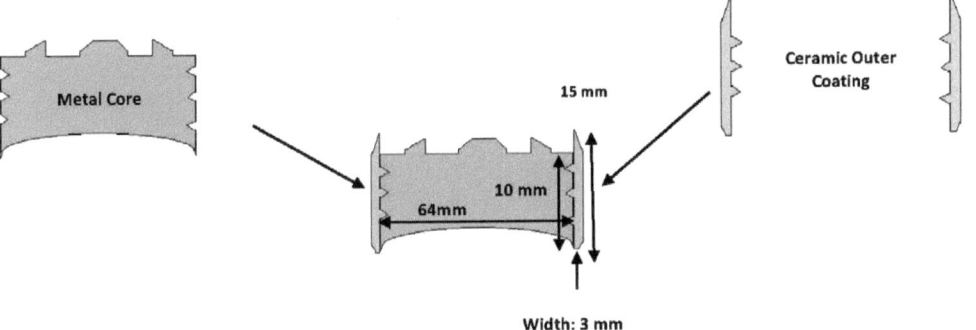

Metal Core

15 mm

10 mm

64mm

Width: 3 mm

Ceramic Outer Coating

Figure 2: Attachment to Vertebra

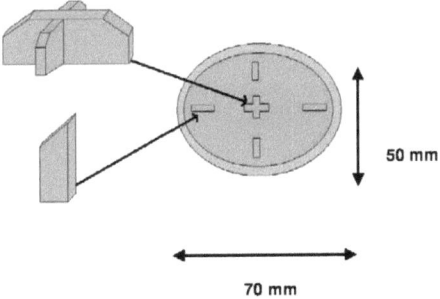

50 mm

70 mm

In the articulating middle piece, which will actually act like the intervertebral disc, an ellipse ultra high molecular weight polyethylene disc with a cone-like silicon elastomer placed in the superio-medial part, as demonstrated in the figure below (Figure 3) is designed.

The ultra high molecular weight polyethylene allows movement because of self-lubricating and low coefficient of friction properties which are essential requirements. The sillicated elastomer is mainly placed to transmit and distribute stress to the elliptic ultra high molecular weight polyethylene disc and prevent surface degradation. Also, the compressible, soft nature of the elastomer allows flexibility and comfort to the patient in movements performed.

Figure 3: Middle Piece

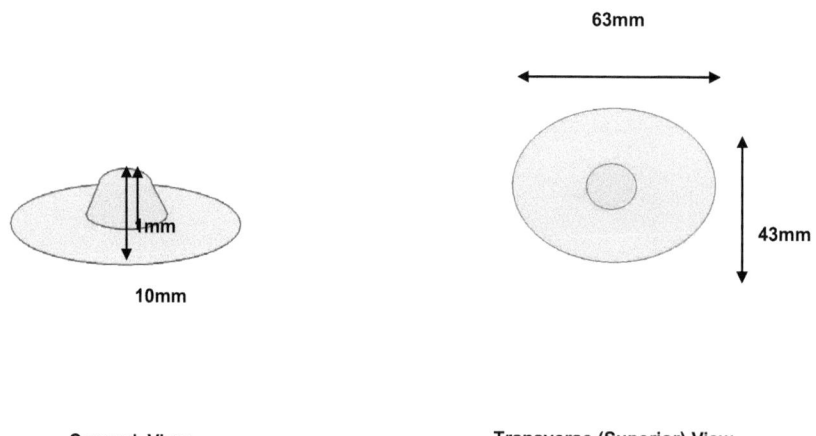

Coronal View   Transverse (Superior) View

The middle piece is attached and locked to the inferior plate. This is because the load is applied from the superior direction and the reaction force is from the inferior direction. In this design, the joint would be more stable.

The combined image for the intervertebral disc replacement product is demonstrated in the figure below (Figure 4).

Figure 4: The Complete Intervertebral Disc Replacement Design

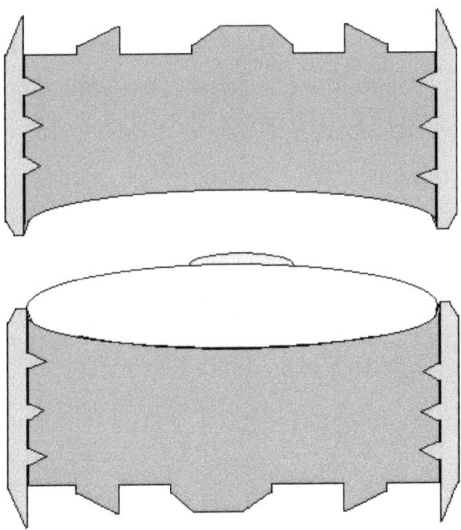

The bone surface will be prepared for the fixation of the replacement device during the operation. The pathological disc, cartilage and probably superficial parts of the bone will be removed, creating space and attachment sites for placement of this designed device. Sometimes, removal of cartilage will not be needed, however attachment sites of the replacement device will reach bone tissue in any condition. A fixator, cement or sticking agent could be used to stabilize the bone-metal attachment.

Replication of intervertebral disc functions as close as possible is an important consideration. The ball and socket joint model is used, with 2 moving parts. This provides a fixed rotation centre and this permits dynamic motion. This mechanism also prevents excessive shear loading on facets.

The arrangement of placement in midline provides a primary fixation. The spiky attachments also distribute stress to different areas of the adjacent bone and the design of spikes makes loosening less prevalent. The ceramics used on sides provide additional fixation. Strong fixation, motion allowance and establishment of balance are essential properties required from an intervertebral disc replacement device and this design addresses these needs successfully.

Testing

The aim of intervertebral disc replacement device design is to replace the human intervertebral disc, and allow painless, stable movement of patients with pathological disc conditions preventing movement in the vertebral range of movement. In order to prove functioning and safety of the product, a series of in-vitro testing methods should be performed.

Static and dynamic properties of design are tested together with the mechanics of the materials. The loading in the in-vitro experiments can never perfectly replicate the in-vivo situation; however, it can give an approximate idea about the success of the design. Fatigue, compression, shear, wear and loading tests should be performed in an attempt to assess the material. Subluxation risk should be tested in shear testing as well. There are viscoelastic parts present in the design so creep and stress relaxation tests should be applied. Cadaveric study for in vivo kinematic testing and determination of movement range in real conditions would be useful. [68]

At least six sample repeats are required for statistic testing and fatigue test.[68] ASTM F2346 proposes some testing protocols for the intervertebral disc replacement products that could be used in this design as well. The conditions for fatigue test are: 0.9%saline solution, 37° temperature and less than or equal to 2Hz rate. These conditions seek reproduction of the environment in human body. Other mediums that can imitate human body could also be used in case of rational justification.[60]

Compression and shear testing are important for determining the safety and functionality in answering the load-bearing requirements. Wear resistance should be tested by wear testing. Clinical assessment of tissue response is also required for observing the debri formation and biocompatibility.

In wear testing, ten million cycles in bovine serum and body temperature are performed as a predictive measure. Controlled load and motion application together with employment of these on the centre of rotation are needed. Both axial and torsional loading would be tested.[61] Axial torsion systems like 8874 servohydraulic and E10000 Electroplus instruments, in body temperature, with addition of recirculator unit, would be used in both static and fatigue testing protocols as well.[62]

Performing these tests in wet environment puts an extra strain on the product. The saline concentration and temperature of the testing are controlled in baths. 8874 testing system allows axial compression, compression-shear and compression-torsion testings for all metal-metal and metal-polyethylene designs.[62] The debris should be extracted from this environment by filtering in every one million cycles and assessed for the increasing or decreasing amount.

The testing must be performed for all flexion, extension, lateral flexion and rotation movements of spine to ensure the patient will be able to perform movements that are originally created by the vertebrae and intervertebral discs. FDA standards for durability and wear tests that would be applied to this design are: 7.5° degree flexion and extension, 6° lateral flexion, 6° axial rotation for cervical vertebra and 3° axial rotation for lumbar vertebra, less than or equal to

2Hz frequency for 10 million cycles with 100N cervical preload or 1200N lumbar preload.[68]

Biocompatibility is an important issue and leachability, molecular weight, weight distribution, structures, crystallinity and cross linking degree would be stated for the polyethylene used in the device. A clinical investigation plan with a designed pilot study with two years or more of follow-up for pain for device failure, ranges of motion, stability of fixation, bone growth, migration of device and amount of fusion needs to be performed. Radiological imaging, gait disturbance, myopathy, and pain information could demonstrate success of the device.[68]

Conclusion

Intervertebral discs are the shock absorbers in the vertebrae and also contribute to the flexibility of spine. Deformation or degradation of these structures could cause pain, nerve compression or gait differences. When the condition gets severe, affecting the cartilage and the bone, a surgery must take place to restore the health of the patient. Intervertebral disc replacement is an option for the surgery. CoCrMo metal plate body with surrounding ceramic coating and an ultra high molecular weight polyethylene middle piece attached to the inferior plate, with an elastomer addition in the middle could be an alternative design for this replacement device.

Acknowledgements

I would like to express my gratitude to the people who helped me to carry out this project. First of all, I would like to express my thankfulness to my teacher Julia Shelton for giving me the opportunity to work on this project as one of my assessments and teaching me very valuable information about the background of this project. I would like to thank Queen Mary, University of London School of Engineering and Materials Science and Barts and the London School of Medicine and Dentistry for providing me the opportunity to perform this work.

I would like to thank my mother Assoc.Prof.Dr.Bahire Efe Özad, my father Ali Ozad, my brother Murat Ozad, my grandmother Ülvan Efe, Musteyde Ozad (late) and, my grandfathers Murad Husnu Ozad (late) and Fadil Efe, for their love, care and support not only during this project, but also throughout my whole life.

References

[1]: W. Arnould-Taylor, A Textbook of Anatomy and Physiology, Pages 16-20, 3rd Edition, 1998, STP.

[2]: J.S. Ross and K.J.W. Wilson, Anatomy and Physiology in Health and Illness, Pages: 12-13, 23-24, 221-225, 246-249,211-315, 6th Edition, 1989, Churchill Livingstone.

[3]: R.L. Drake et al, Gray's Anatomy for Students, Pages 57-59, 2nd Edition, 2010, Churchill Livingstone.

[4]: K.L. Moore and A.M.R Agur, Essential Clinical Anatomy, Page 272, 3rd Edition, 2007, Lippincott Williams and Wilkins.

[5]:K.L. Moore et al, Clinically Oriented Anatomy, Page 442-464, 6th Edition, 2010, Lippincott Williams and Wilkins.

[6]: Omar Faiz & David Moffat. Anatomy at a Glance. 2nd Ed. Blackwell Publishing, 2006.

[7]: H.Marieb, Human Anatomy and Physiology, Page 217, 2009, 8th Edition, Benjamin Cummings.

[8]: Vertebra and Spinal Nerves, Health Central, A.D.A.M, Online Resource, Last Accessed: 08 December 2011 12:33, http://www.healthcentral.com/osteoporosis/9936-146.html.

[9]: Intervertebral Discs, Spine Universe, Online Resource, Last Accessed: 08 December 2011 13:29, http://www.spineuniverse.com/anatomy/intervertebral-discs.

[10]: R.Rokhamm, Colour Atlas of Neurology, Page 30, 2004, Thieme.

[11]: F.H. Netter, Atlas of Human Anatomy, Page 155, 4th Edition, 2006, Saunders.

[12]: The internal mechanical properties of cervical intervertebral discs as revealed by stress profilometry, Daniel M. Skrzypiec,2 Phillip Pollintine,1 Andrzej Przybyla,3 Patricia Dolan,1 and Michael A. Adams1 1Department of Anatomy, University of Bristol, Southwell Street, Bristol, BS2 8EJ UK, 2Section of Biomechanics, Hamburg University of Technology, Hamburg, Germany, 3Biomechanics Group, Penn State University, Harrisburg, PA USA.

[13]: New In Vivo Measurements of Pressures in the Intervertebral Disc in Daily Life, Hans–Joachim Wilke, PhD, Peter Neef, MD, Marco Caimi, MD, Thomas Hoogland, MD and Lutz E. Claes, PhD.

[14]: Peak stresses observed in the posterior lateral anulus. Edwards WT, Ordway NR, Zheng Y, McCullen G, Han Z, Yuan HA. Department of Physical Medicine and Rehabilitation, SUNY Upstate Medical University, Syracuse, NY 13210, US.

[15]: 'STRESS' DISTRIBUTIONS INSIDE INTERVERTEBRAL DISCS THE EFFECTS OF AGE AND DEGENERATION, M. A. ADAMS, D. S. MCNALLY, P. DOLAN, From the University of Bristol, England.

[16]: S. Roberts and J.P.G. Urban, Intervertebral Discs, Online Resource, Last Accessed: 8 December 2011 14:41, http://www.ilo.org/safework_bookshelf/english?content&nd=857170059.

[17]: Back pain, BUPA, Online Resource, Last Accessed: 08 December 2011 19:43, http://www.bupa.co.uk/individuals/health-information/directory/b/backpain.

[18]: V.C. Scanlon and T.Sanders, Essentials of Anatomy and Physiology, Pages 120-123, 5th Edition, 2007, F.A.Davis.

[19]: E.G.Dawson, Herniated Discs: Definition, Progression, and Diagnosis, Spine Universe, Online Resource, Last Accessed: 08 December 2011 20:12, http://www.spineuniverse.com/conditions/herniated-disc/herniated-discs-definition-progression-diagnosis.

[20]: Prolapsed Disc, Patient.co.uk, Online Resource, Last Accessed: 08 December 2011 20:24, http://www.patient.co.uk/health/Prolapsed-Disc-%28Slipped-Disc%29.htm.

[21]: C.D. Ray, Osteoarthritis of the Spine, Spine-Health, Online Resource, Last Accessed: 08 December 2011 22:55, http://www.spine-health.com/conditions/arthritis/osteoarthritis-spine.

[22]: P. Kumar and M. Clark. Kumar and Clark Clinical Medicine, 6th Edition, 2005, Elsevier Saunders.

[23]: C. Eustice, Spine Osteoarthritis, About.com, Online Resource, Last Accessed: 08 December 2011 23:12, http://osteoarthritis.about.com/od/spinespinalosteoarthritis/a/spine_OA.htm.

[24]: Radiological Degenerative Joint Disease (Osteoarthritis) of the Spine, Online Resource, Last Accessed: 8 December 2011 23:45, http://www.glucosamine-arthritis.org/arthritis/DJD-Spine.html.

[25]: Osteoarthritis of the Spine, eMedicine Health, Online Resource, Last Accessed: 8 December 2011 23:48, http://www.emedicinehealth.com/script/main/art.asp?articlekey=138825&ref=128218.

[26]: Centers for Medicare and Medicaid Services, Online Resource, Last Accessed: 09 December 2011 08:57, http://www.cms.hhs.gov/EOG/downloads/EO%200051.pdf.

[27]: AA Patel et al., Revision Strategies for Lumbar Total Disc Arthroplasty, Spine, 33(11):1276-83, 15 May 2008.

[28]: NICE, Online Resource, Last Accessed: 9 December 2011 09:44, http://www.nice.org.uk/.

[29]: Normal Human Range of Motion, Livestrong, Online resource, Last Accessed: 11 December 2011 09:56, http://www.livestrong.com/article/257162-normal-human-range-of-motion/.

[30]: Spine Biomechanics- A brief Overview, BME 456, 2011, Michigan Engineering School.

[31]: Spinal Fusion, Encyclopedia of Surgery, Online Resource, Last Accessed: 11 December 2011 10:14, http://www.surgeryencyclopedia.com/Pa-St/Spinal-Fusion.html.

[32]: Sterilization, Infection Prevention Guidelines, Perkins JJ. 1983. Principles and Methods of Sterilization in Health Sciences, 2nd ed. Charles C. Thomas Publisher Ltd.: Springfield, IL, pp

95–166; 286–311.

[33]: Martz, E. O., Lakes, R. S., Goel, V. K. and Park, J. B. "Design of an artificial intervertebral disc exhibiting a negative Poisson's ratio", Cellular Polymers, 24, 127-138, (2005).

[34]: Prosthetic intervertebral disc replacement in the lumbar spine, NICE, Online resource, last Accessed: 21 November 2011 11:34, http://www.nice.org.uk/IPG306.

[35]: S. Taksali et al, Material considerations for intervertebral disc replacement implants, The Spine Journal
Volume 4, Issue 6, Supplement, November-December 2004, Pages S231-S238.

[36]: J.B. Park and J.D. Bronzino, Biomaterials Principles and Applications, Pages 3-15, 85,160,170, 2003, CRC Press.

[37]:Semlitsch, 1980, Retrieved from: J.B. Park and J.D. Bronzino, Biomaterials Principles and Applications, Pages 3-5, 2003, CRC Press.

[38]: American Society For Testing Materials, F75- Page 42, F562- Page 150, 1992.

[39]: Implants, Randall Dryer, Online Resource, Last Accessed: 11 December 2011 13:01, http://www.artificial-disc-surgery.com/Implants.htm.

[40]: American Society for Testing Materials, page 36-84, 1992 and Davidson et al., 1994 Retrieved from: J.B. Park and J.D. Bronzino, Biomaterials Principles and Applications, Pages 3-5, 2003, CRC Press.

[41]: Neurosurgical Instruments, Online Resource, Last Accessed: 11 December 2011 13:32, http://www.neurocirugia.com/instrumental/index.php?category=34.

[42]: Innovasive Materials, Julisch, Online Resource, Last Accessed: 11 December 2011 13:33, http://www.fz-juelich.de/iek/iek-1/EN/Research/Werkstoffe/WST_Artikel.html.

[43]: Astell, Online Resource, Last Accessed: 21 November 2011 19:01, http://www.astell.com/sterilizer.

[44]: G.P.Jacobs, Radiation Sterilization of Parenterals, 1 May 2007, Online Resource, Last Accessed: 21 November 2011 19:09,

http://pharmtech.findpharma.com/pharmtech/Aseptic+Processing/Radiation-Sterilization-of-Parenterals/ArticleStandard/Article/detail/423948.

[45]: American Society for Testing Materials, page 61-86, 1992, Retrieved from: J.B. Park and J.D. Bronzino, Biomaterials Principles and Applications, Pages 3-5, 2003, CRC Press.

[46]: The Spine Institute, Online Resource, Last Accessed: 21 November 2011 20:58, http://www.laspineinstitute.com/artificialdiscreplacement.htm[24]: ASTM F2346-05, Online Resource, Last Accessed: 21 November 2011 20:56, http://www.astm.org/Standards/F2346.htm.

[47]: Specimen Preparation and Spine Conditions, Medscape, Online resource, Last Accessed: 11 December 2011 17:17, http://www.medscape.com/viewarticle/489864_2.

[48]: Spinal Disc Replacement, Spine Universe, Online Resource, Last Accessed: 11 December 2011 18:07, http://www.spineuniverse.com/treatments/emerging/artificial-discs/spinal-disc-replacement-development-artificial.

[49]: Elastomer Properties Chart, JCB, Online Resource, Last Accessed: 21 November 2011 19:15, http://www.jgbhose.com/Data_Returns/rubber.asp.

[50]: J.B. Park and J.D. Bronzino, Biomaterials Principles and Applications, Pages 60-80, 1992, CRC Press.

[51]: Materials used in Orthopaedic Implants, Zimmer, Online Resource, Last Accessed: 18 November 2011 19:14, www.zimmer.com/ctl?template=PC&op=global&action=1&id=9480.

[52]: The Spine Institute, Online Resource, Last Accessed: 21 November 2011 20:58, http://www.laspineinstitute.com/artificialdiscreplacement.htm[24]: ASTM F2346-05, Online Resource, Last Accessed: 21 November 2011.

[53]: Orthopedic Implant and Orthotic Applications, Ticona, Online Resource, Last Accessed: 17 November 2011 19:58, http://www.ticona.com/home_page/markets/medical/orthopedic_implant_and_orthotic_applications.htm.

[54]: B.D.Ratner et al, Biomaterials Science, Pages 67-170, 2004, Second Edition, Elsevier.

[55]: Cervical Cage, Scient'x, Online Resource, Last Accessed: 20 December 2011 22:21, http://www.biorad-medisys.com/samarys_&_CBK_cervical_cage.html.

[56]: M Filip et al., Replacement of an intervertebral disc, using a ceramic prosthesis, in the treatment of degenerative diseases of the spine, Acta Chir Orthop Traumatol Cech. 1995;62(4):226-31.

[57]: S.S.Block, Disinfection, Sterilization and Preservation, 2nd Edition, 1977, Lea and Febiger.

[58]: S. Umehara et al., Effects of degeneration on the elastic modulus distribution in the lumbar intervertebral disc, Spine (Phila Pa 1976). 1996 Apr 1;21(7):811-9; discussion 820.

[59]: ProDisc L Total Disc Replacement, Synthes Spine, Online Resource, Last Accessed: 15 November 2011 20:15, http://www.synthes.com/MediaBin/US%20DATA/Product%20Support%20Mat erials/Technique%20Guides/SPINE/SPTGProDisc-LJ6206D.pdf.

[60]: ASTM F2346-05, Online Resource, Last Accessed: 21 November 2011 20:56, http://www.astm.org/Standards/F2346.htm.

[61]: Testing, medscape, Online resource, Last Accessed: 12 December 2011 23:55, http://www.medscape.com/viewarticle/495415_4.

[62]: Characterization and Fatigue of Spinal Intervertebral Body Fusion Devices (ASTM F2077), Instron, Online Resource, Last Accessed: 13 December 2011 00.00, http://www.instron.co.uk/wa/solutions/ASTM-F2077-

Fatigue-Testing-Spinal-Intervertebral-Body-Fusion-Devices.aspx?ref=http://www.google.co.uk/url.

[63]: Characterization and Fatigue of Intervertebral Disc Prostheses, Instron, Online Resource, Last Accessed: 21 November 2011 20:59, http://www.instron.co.uk/wa/solutions/ASTM-F2346-Fatigue-Artifical-Spinal-Discs.aspx?ref=http://www.google.co.uk/url.

[64]: Herniated Nucleus Pulposus, Medscape, Online resource, Last Accessed: 12 December 2011 22:29, http://emedicine.medscape.com/article/1263961-overview.

[65]: Cartilage Types, Online resource, Last Accessed: 12 December 2011 22:46, http://www.vetmed.vt.edu/education/curriculum/vm8054/labs/Lab7/lab7.htm.

[66]: What is Intervertebral Disc Degeneration, and What Causes It?: Disc Functional Anatomy, Medscape, Online Resource, Last Accessed: 12 December 2011 23:05, http://www.medscape.com/viewarticle/543611_2 and spine, 2006 Lippincott Williams and Wilkins.

[67]: A.J. Peacock, Handbook of Polyethylene – Structures, Properties and Applications, Pages 1-7, 2000, Marcel Decker.

[68]: Guidance for Industry and FDA Staff: Preparation and Review of Investigational Device Exemption Applications (IDEs) for Total Artificial Discs, FDA, Online Resource, Last Accessed: 14 December 2011 09:52, http://www.fda.gov/medicaldevices/deviceregulationandguidance/guidancedocuments/ucm071154.htm.

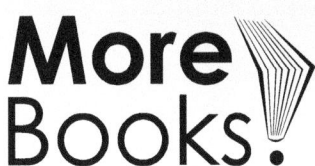
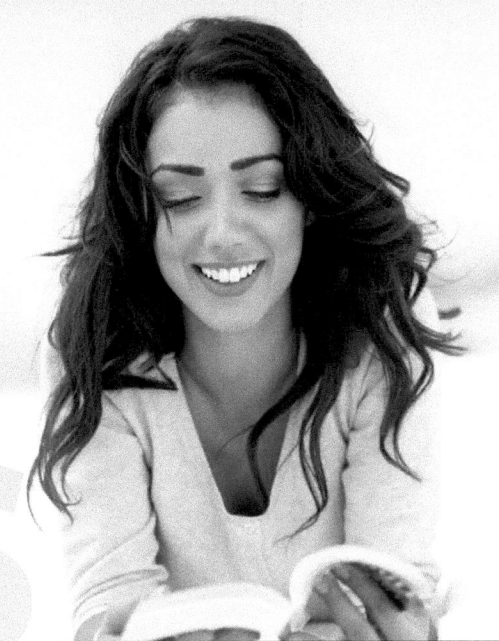
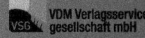

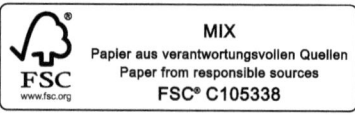